YOUR KNOWLEDGE HAS VALUE

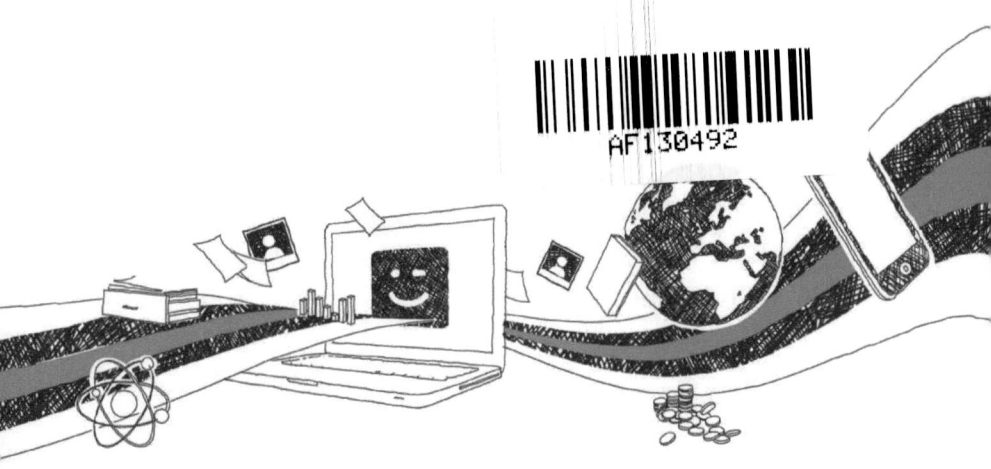

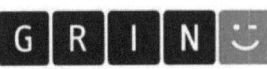

Clavicle Fractures. Clinical Picture, Diagnosis, Treatment

Raveendran Gokul

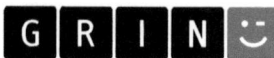

Bibliographic information published by the German National Library:

The German National Library lists this publication in the National Bibliography; detailed bibliographic data are available on the Internet at http://dnb.dnb.de.

ISBN: 9783389032152
This book is also available as an ebook.

© GRIN Publishing GmbH
Trappentreustraße 1
80339 München

Print and binding: Books on Demand GmbH, Norderstedt, Germany
Printed on acid-free paper from responsible sources.

The present work has been carefully prepared. Nevertheless, authors and publishers do not incur liability for the correctness of information, notes, links and advice as well as any printing errors.

GRIN web shop: https://www.grin.com/document/1475764

Ministry of Health of the Republic of Moldova

Nicolae Testemiţanu State University of Medicine and Pharmacy

FACULTY OF MEDICINE 2

Department of **Orthopedics & traumatology**

Graduation Thesis

CLAVICLE FRACTURES: CLINICAL PICTURE, DIAGNOSIS, TREATMENT

RAVEENDRAN NAIR BEENA GOKUL

Year VI, group 1877

Study program 0912.1 Medicine

Chisinau, 2024

CONTENTS

LIST OF ABBREVATIONS

ACJ - Acromioclavicular joint

AO - Association of Osteosynthesis

AP-Antero-Posterior

CA-Coracoacromial

CT - Computed tomography

CF – Clavicular fracture

IM - Intramuscular

ORIF - Open reduction and internal fixation

SCM - Sternocleidomastoid muscle

INTRODUCTION

The actuality of the research

Clavicle fractures usually affect people under the age of 25, with children and young adults suffering from them the most frequently. The clavicle is a common area for injury due to its superficial placement, its thin midshaft, and the pressures transmitted across it. A hard fall with the arm at the side, which frequently happens during contact sports, is the most frequent mechanism of injury. The history and physical examination can frequently make a diagnosis, but suitable radiography should be done to confirm the diagnosis and provide treatment options. The majority of midshaft clavicle fractures can be managed nonoperatively. Children frequently have significant calluses, so parents may need assurance.[22]

Surgery is an option for fractures with a high risk of nonunion (e.g., displaced or comminuted fractures, fractures with more than 15 to 20 mm clavicle shortening). The relationship of the distal fracture to the coracoclavicular ligaments determines the likelihood of displacement.[17]

The aim of the thesis:

- To investigate theoretical data (classification, epidemiology, symptoms, treatment, complications) in order to improve the knowledge and management of clavicle fracture and to analyze the clinical data of the patients with CFs treated in the Department of traumatology nr.1, Institute of Emergency Medicine, during the years 2019-2023.

Objectives of the thesis:

1. To review the anatomy and biomechanics of the clavicle and the mechanisms of clavicle fractures.
2. To investigate the incidence, classification and clinical presentation and diagnostic of clavicle fractures, treatment methods according to the type of fracture.
3. To perform a retrospective and prospective study of the patients with CFs treated in the Department of traumatology nr.1, Institute of Emergency Medicine, during the years 2019-2023.
4. To analyze the diagnostic & treatment methods applied to the patients with clavicle fractures.

1. CLAVICLE FRACTURES (LITERATURE REVIEW)

1.1. Anatomy of the clavicle

1.1.1. Bone structure.

This image has been removed for copyright reasons.

Figure 1:Anatomy of clavicle[57]

The clavicle is a long bone. It provides shoulder support, allowing the arm to swing freely away from the trunk. The weight of the limb is transferred from the clavicle to the sternum. The bone has a cylindrical part called the shaft, and it has two ends, lateral and medial.[35]

Side Determination

The following characters indicate which side of the body a clavicle belongs to:

1. Lateral end- flat, the medial end- large and quadrilateral.
2. The shaft has a little curvature, with its medial two-thirds convex and its lateral one-third concave.
3. A longitudinal groove runs through the middle third of the inferior surface.[3]

Clavicle Distinctions

- It is the only horizontally oriented long bone.
- It lies subcutaneously.
- It is the initial bone to begin ossification.
- It is the only long bone that forms a membrane ossification.
- It is the only long bone with two ossification primary centers.
- The medullary cavity is absent.
- It is occasionally pierced by the middle supraclavicular nerve.[45]

Features

Shaft. There are two halves to the shaft: the medial two-thirds and the lateral one-third. Due to its subcutaneous, more anterior placement, and frequent exposure to transmitted stresses, the clavicle is prone to fracture easily. Because it lacks muscle and ligamentous support, the middle third, also known as the midshaft, is the thinnest and least medullous part of the clavicle and is hence most prone to fractures. Strong ligamentous and capsular support underpins the sternoclavicular (SC) and acromioclavicular (AC) joints. The sternal ossification center of the clavicle completes ossification and fuses with the shaft by 30 years of age.[10]

Eighty percent of the bone's longitudinal growth is attributed to this medial ossification region. Adolescents with open growth plates should be evaluated for potential physical injury. The clavicle is a long bone with a sigmoid shape and a convex surface along its medial end when viewed from the cephalad position.[28]

Clavicle connects the axial and appendicular skeletons, as well as the scapula, and these structures form the pectoral girdle.

1.1.2 Ligaments

Attachment on clavicle /Collarbone	Ligaments	Other attachments
Inferior surface	Trapezoid ligament (the lateral part of the coracoclavicular ligament)	Trapezoid line
Inferior surface	Conoid ligament (the medial part of the coracoclavicular ligament)	Conoid tubercle

1.1.3. Muscles

There are various muscular attachments on the clavicle that need to be taken into account anatomically. Superior surface: The anterior deltoid muscle originates on the anterior aspect and facilitates shoulder flexion, conversely, the posterior portion contains one of the trapezius muscle's insertion sites. Stabilization of the scapula is mostly the responsibility of the trapezius.[38]

·   Inferior surface: The subclavius muscle pulls the clavicle anteroinferiorly and depresses the shoulder. It is situated in the clavicle's subclavian groove. The coracoid, which is situated below, is supported by the coracoacromial ligament, which is lateral. The conoid ligament, which attaches to the conoid tubercle, forms the medial component of the CA ligament, while the trapezoid ligament, which attaches to the trapezoid line, forms the lateral component.

·   Anterior surface: The medial clavicle serves as the anterior source for the clavicular segment of the pectoralis major muscle. The bending of the humerus, horizontal adduction, and inward rotation are made easier by the clavicular head.

·   Posterior surface: As mentioned before, the trapezius inserts on the clavicle postero-superiorly. Along the medial third of the clavicle is also where the clavicular head of the sternocleidomastoid (SCM) is situated. The ipsilateral side bends laterally and the head turns to the other side when the SCM contracts on its own. The head flexes when the SCM contracts together.[41]

This image has been removed for copyright reasons.

Figure 2:Muscles and ligaments surrounding clavicle[56]

1.1.4. *Vascularization*

The clavicle, unlike other long bones, lacks a medullary cavity even though it is categorized as a long bone. Prior studies have demonstrated that the bone structure possesses a periosteal arterial blood supply, but not a central nutrient artery. It has been found that the clavicle receives vascular flow from the thoracoacromial artery, internal thoracic artery (mammalian artery), and suprascapular artery.[46]

1.1.5. Nerves

There is disagreement over the clavicle's major sensory innervation. Research on anesthesia following clavicular fractures has indicated that the long thoracic/suprascapular n., subclavian nerve (n.), and supraclavicular nerve (n.) may be linked. One common anatomical variation is a perforating branch of the supraclavicular n. that enters through the superior surface of the clavicle. Exams performed after death have shown that nerves are inserted into bony tunnels or grooves which are vulnerable to injury, and could account for entrapment neuropathy after clavicular fractures.[13]

1.2. Classification of clavicle fractures

When evaluating clavicular fractures, one of the most widely used classification methods is the AO classification.[4]

AO classification

This image has been removed for copyright reasons.

Figure 3:AO Classification system for clavicle fractures[54]

The AO classification of clavicle fracture is a system used to categorize clavicle fractures based on their location and severity. It is a commonly used classification scheme that aids medical professionals in choosing the most appropriate course of action for every given situation.[42]

Three primary categories are distinguished by the AO classification for clavicle fractures:

Type A

Type A = nondisplaced + intact Coracoclavicular ligaments

Type A: Extra-articular fractures

- A1: Fracture of the lateral third of the clavicle

- A2: Fracture of the middle third of the clavicle

- A3: Fracture of the medial third of the clavicle

Type B

Type B = displaced + intact Coracoclavicular ligaments

Type B: Partially articular fractures

- B1: Fracture of the lateral third of the clavicle involving the acromioclavicular joint

- B2: Fracture of the medial third of the clavicle involving the sternoclavicular joint

Type C

Type C = displaced + torn Coracoclavicular ligaments

Type C: Completely articular fractures

- C1: Fracture of the lateral third of the clavicle involving the acromioclavicular joint and coracoclavicular ligament

- C2: Fracture of the middle third of the clavicle involving the acromioclavicular joint and coracoclavicular ligament

- C3: Fracture of the medial third of the clavicle involving the sternoclavicular joint and/or the first rib

1.3. Mechanism of clavicle fractures

A fall onto the shoulder is responsible for about 87% of clavicle fractures.[12] The majority of fractures in young people are caused by sports and traffic accidents . Bicyclists suffer 39% of injuries from traffic accidents, followed by drivers or passengers of cars (26%), pedestrians (17%), and motorcyclists (17%).[32][37]

A direct impact from an item to the clavicle (7%) and indirect trauma from falls onto an outstretched hand (6%) are unusual causes of clavicle fractures . The fracture site (i.e., which third is damaged) and the method of injury are unrelated [31].

1.4. Clinical picture of the clavicle fractures

Clavicle fractures are usually easy to be found due to the superficial localization of the collarbone. The most common clinical signs of the CF are:

- Pain
- Sagging of the shoulder downward and forward[48]
- Inability to lift the arm because of pain
- A grinding sensation when trying to raise the arm
- A deformity or bump over the break. The superior displacement of the medial fragment seen in midshaft fractures could be due to SCM tension, which could lead to further instability.[29]
- Bruising, swelling, and/or tenderness over the collarbone
- Forced "antalgic" position
- It is rare for a bone fragment to break through the skin, it may push the skin into a tent formation[27]

10% of all fractures are clavicle fractures, which are the most dangerous kind of collarbone injury.[5] Depending on comminution, displacement, and shortening, surgery can be required. SCM stress may be the cause of the superior displacement of the medial fragment observed in midshaft fractures, which could result in further instability. 87% of the time, trauma—like a fall that strikes the shoulder laterally—is the source of the injury.[26][50] Other possible causes of the injury include falling outward onto an extended hand or making medial contact with the clavicle.[1]

10

1.5. Diagnosis of clavicle fractures

A standard anteroposterior clavicle radiograph should be done of any patient who presents with a clavicle injury. The evaluation of the degree of clavicle dislocation is improved by a second radiograph featuring a 45-degree cephalic tilt view. The scapula and first rib overlap is further lessened by this extra viewpoint. Although the majority of clavicle fractures are visible in these views, a CT scan may be necessary to determine whether intra-articular involvement exists in the less common proximal or distal fractures and to guide treatment. A pneumothorax or rib injury should be clinically suspected, and this can be confirmed with an expiratory posteroanterior chest radiograph. If neurovascular damage is suspected, arteriography, ultrasonography, and CT may be utilized to direct further treatment.[9]

A CT scan and plain radiography images are utilized to assess proximal clavicular stress fractures, if necessary. To rule out inflammation and neoplasia in individuals exhibiting both radiographic and clinical signs of edema surrounding this location, more imaging tests could be necessary.[24]

This image has been removed for copyright reasons.

Figure 4:CT image of a clavicle fracture[56]

X-ray. An isolated anteroposterior (AP) projection focused on the midshaft of the clavicle is observed in fractures of the middle third of the clavicle, and radiography is typically the only modality needed. If there is a significant level of clinical suspicion and the AP view does not show a fracture, a 30° cephalic view may be helpful. The following findings could be made:

- A clavicular fracture is most commonly found at the junction of the lateral and middle thirds of the clavicle.
- A greenstick fracture, or incomplete fracture, can happen in kids.
- Newborns may sustain clavicle fractures during tough deliveries.
- The medial clavicular fragment is usually cranially displaced due to the pull of the sternocleidomastoid muscle.
- Most cases involve both an acromio-clavicular joint dislocation and a clavicle fracture, which are typically mutually exclusive.[6]

This image has been removed for copyright reasons.

Figure 5:X-ray image of a fracture of distal third part of clavicle [55]

1.6. Complications of the clavicle fractures

The two most frequent complications of proximal clavicle fractures are posttraumatic arthritis and nonunion. Pneumothorax, subclavian venous laceration, and compression of the brachial plexus are among the serious injuries that can arise from inward sternoclavicular dislocations or fracture fragments. [2]

- The most frequent consequence of clavicle fractures is malunion, which occurs when the fracture heals with angulation, shortening, or an unfavorable look. The majority of patients with clavicle fracture malunion are clinically inconsequential and have full function. Certain malunions, particularly those with a shortening of more than 2 cm, may result in neurological or functional problems. Patients with persistent discomfort, limited range of motion, or diminished strength due to a malunion may benefit from a delayed surgical repair.[16]

- When a fracture doesn't heal in four to six months, it's called nonunion. In middle-third clavicle fractures treated nonoperatively, the nonunion rate is 6%; in displaced fractures, it rises to 15%. The nonunion rate for fractures of the distal third clavicle varies from 28% to 44%. Risk factors for nonunion include advanced age, female gender, smoking, fracture comminution, considerable displacement or shortening of the fracture, and insufficient immobilization. Many people with nonunion clavicle fractures are asymptomatic and don't need any additional care. Some individuals may have persistent pain, limited range of motion, or loss of function due to symptomatic clavicle fracture nonunion. These individuals should be sent to an orthopedic specialist for additional surgical care.[15]
- Clavicle fractures rarely result in serious consequences. Injury to the brachial plexus or subclavian vessels might happen during presentation or when the clavicle heals and forms a callus. Peripheral neuropathy may arise from brachial plexus compression brought on by excessive callus production.[21]
- Two complications of fractures to the proximal-third clavicle include nonunion and posttraumatic arthritis. Internally displaced proximal clavicle fractures can result in serious intrathoracic injuries such pneumothorax, brachial plexus injury, and subclavian artery injury. The highest rate of nonunion occurs in the distal third of clavicle fractures; nevertheless, many of these patients' nonunion are asymptomatic. Degenerative arthritis of the articuloclavicular joint is a late consequence.[7]

1.7. Treatment of clavicle fractures

Depending on a number of variables, including position (mid-shaft, distal, proximal), nature (displaced, undisplaced, comminuted), open versus closed injury, age, and neurovascular impairments, clavicle fractures are treated surgically or conservatively.[39][49]

1.7.1. Conservative treatment

A conservative approach to treating clavicle fractures has involved immobilization with a sling and after-care rehabilitation. Conservative treatment of displaced mid-shaft clavicle fractures leads to thoracoscapular dyskinesia, prolonged recovery periods for returning to sport, and suboptimal shoulder function as a result of clavicular mal-union and shortening. Similarly, it has been demonstrated that athletes with displaced lateral fractures who get conservative care have significant rates of non-union and consequent reduction of shoulder function.[8]

1.7.1.1Nonoperative treatment of clavicle fractures

Phase 1: injury until the third week following the injury (inflammatory phase) (inflammatory phase)

Phase 1 principle: protection of the injured (operated) limb to facilitate uneventful healing.

Phase 1 aim: healing without complications while facilitating early movement.[23]

External support - full time

When the forearm and upper arm are fastened to the chest, the shoulder is immobilized as effectively as possible. This has traditionally been accomplished with a sling that balances the arm's weight and supports the elbow and forearm. The most basic sling consists of a triangle bandage fastened behind the neck.[20]

A swath that encircles the chest and humerus to prevent further shoulder mobility and maintain the arm safely in the sling offers extra support.[30]

This figure has been removed for copyright reasons.

Figure 6:External support - full time with sling[53]

Abduction brace

When a person has rotator cuff surgery or an acromial or coracoid fracture, they try to decompress by elevating and abducing the affected limb. An abduction cushion, often known as a "airplane splint," can help achieve this.[44]

This figure has been removed for copyright reasons.

Figure 7:Abduction brace[53]

Upper extremity mobilization for general indications

To minimize arm swelling, it is crucial to preserve maximum range of motion in the unaffected joints by promoting lymphatic drainage and venous return. Proprioception is preserved when the unaffected joints are actively mobilized, which facilitates ideal joint motion.

The recommended exercises are as follows.

- Opening and closure of the hand
- Squeezing of a soft ball

This figure has been removed for copyright reasons.

Figure 8:Squeezing of a soft ball[53]

- Bending of the wrist forward, backwards and in a circular motion.
- Movement of an open hand from side to side

This figure has been removed for copyright reasons.

Figure 9:Hand movement exercise[53]

- Straightening and bending of the elbow
- Squeezing the shoulder blades together while the shoulders remain relaxed
- Gentle side-to-side, forward-and-backward, and rotational movements of the neck

Phase 2: Week four to week six following injury (early repair phase)

Phase 2 principle: continued protection of the injured (operated) limb with the promotion of directed tissue repair.

Phase 2 aim: established healing of injured tissues with antigravity strength

Phase 3: After injury, from the start of week 7 until the end of week 12 (late repair and early tissue remodeling phase)

Phase 3 principle: reestablishment of proprioception in the limb.

Phase 3 aim: through regular activities, promote normal tissue structure and reinnervation without causing further harm.

Phase 4: Beginning of the thirteenth week following the injury (remodeling and reintegration phase)

Phase 4 principle: normalization of the proprioceptive function with optimal biomechanics

Phase 4 aim: to establish normal tissue structure and reinnervation through training and practice for optimal endurance.

1.7.2. Surgical treatment
Operative management of clavicular fractures is indicated by:
- Significant displacement brought on by comminution, accompanied with angulation and tenting of the skin that is not responsive to closed reduction and poses a threat to its integrity.
- Neurovascular impairment brought on by a symptomatic shoulder girdle non-union.
- Neurovascular compromise or progressive injury that does not improve after the fracture has healed.
- Multiple traumas, where patient movement is sought and closed methods of immobilization are problematic or not practicable.[25]
- Open fractures.

- Type 2 distal clavicular fractures.
- Incapacity to sustain closed immobilization, such as Parkinson's illness or seizure disorders;
- floating shoulder;
- cosmetic purpose;
- Relative indicators include displacement larger than the clavicle's breadth and shortening of more than 15 to 20 mm.[47][51]

Surgical procedures include:

1. Open reduction and internal fixation (ORIF): This surgical procedure involves making an incision over the fracture site and realigning the broken bone fragments. The fragments are then held in place with metal plates and screws until the bone heals.[33][43]

This figure has been removed for copyright reasons.

Figure 10:Hook plate for Lateral, displaced fracture with CC disrupted, articular clavicle fracture[53]

This figure has been removed for copyright reasons.

Figure 11:The hook plate is secured to the shaft fragment with cortical and cancellous screws [53]

2. Intramedullary fixation: This procedure involves inserting a metal rod through the center of the clavicle to stabilize the fracture. The rod is secured in place with screws at each end.[11][19]

3. Percutaneous fixation: This minimally invasive procedure involves inserting small metal pins through the skin and into the bone to hold the fracture in place.[36][14]

18

4. Plate fixation: This involves attaching a metal plate to the surface of the clavicle using screws to hold the bone fragments in place while they heal.[18]

This figure has been removed for copyright reasons.

Figure 12:Compression plate for
Diaphyseal simple, transverse clavicle fracture[53]

This figure has been removed for copyright reasons.

Figure 13:Compression plate for
Diaphyseal simple, transverse clavicle fracture in place[53]

The choice of surgical procedure depends on the severity and location of the fracture, as well as the patient's age, activity level, and overall health.

In cases of midshaft displaced fractures, metalwork removal was recommended for IM nails but not for plate fixation.[52] While routine removal of hardware was performed for screw, cerclage wire, tension band, and "hook" plate fixation, it was not performed for suture and "non-ACJ-spanning" plate fixation in cases involving displaced lateral clavicle fractures. These fixing procedures are required for lateral clavicle fractures because they include the acromioclavicular joint and multiple ligaments that may be injured during fracture.[34][40]

2.MATERIAL AND METHOD OF RESEARCH

A study was carried out using the clinical records of 94 patients who received treatment for clavicle fractures at the Institute of Emergency Medicine's Department of Traumatology, Nr 1.

Details such as age, gender, trauma etiology, length of hospital stay, treatment options, and other information were gathered from the hospital archive. Following statistical processing using Microsoft Office software, all of the data were put into visual representations.

The study's data was gathered between January 1, 2019, and December 31, 2023. A total of 94 patients' histories were examined for this.

The following is the distribution broken down by year:

❖ 2019 - ...11
❖ 2020 - ...21
❖ 2021 - ...17
❖ 2022- ...21
❖ 2023- ...24

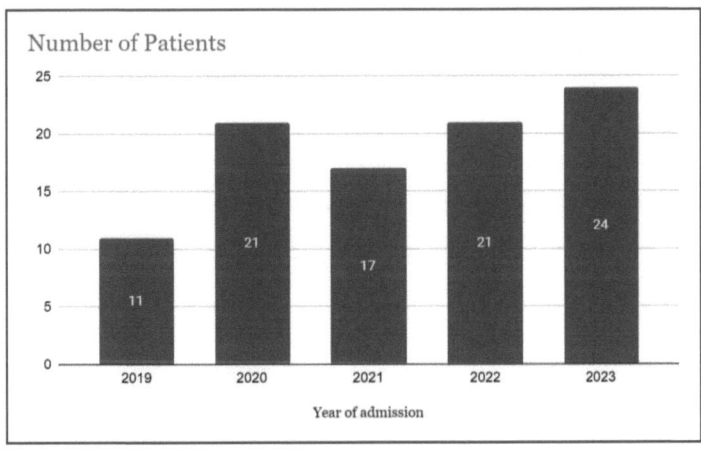

Figure 14. Distribution by the year of admission

There were 21 female patients and 73 male patients(figure 15). This led us to the conclusion that whilst 22.3% of patients with clavicular fractures were female, 77.7% of patients were male. These results allow us to conclude that male sex may be a risk factor for clavicle fractures.

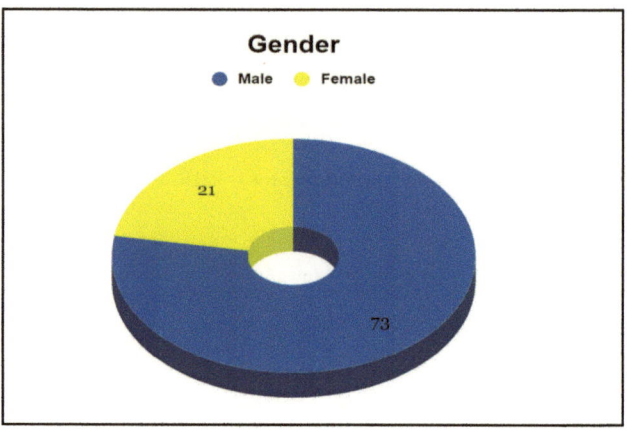

Fig 15.Female-male ratio in clavicular fracture incidence

Age distribution.

We may clearly deduce from the study's findings that the incidence of clavicle fractures rises with advancing age. It was discovered that in the allotted time, just 20 patients under the age of 25 had been admitted to the hospital. The likelihood of a fracture also rises with age. As a result, 51 cases fell into the 26–45 age range, whereas 11 cases fell into the 46–60 age range. Out of 94 instances, 12 were found to be after the age of 60. The majority of individuals in the 26–45 age group had fractures to their clavicles.

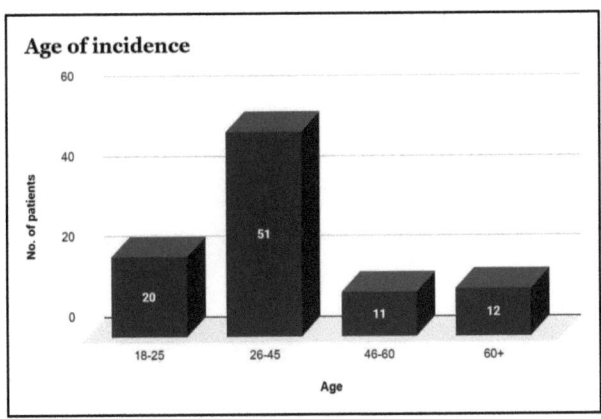

Figure 16.Age distribution graph for clavicle fractures

Cause of Trauma

Trauma at home, trauma at work, sports, and road accidents are the main causes of clavicle fractures. This study shows that habitual trauma affects the majority of the admitted patients. Among the 94 patients, 1.1% had experienced trauma from sports, 20.2% had been in a road accident, 20.2% had experienced trauma at home, 2.1% had experienced trauma at work, and 56.4% had experienced habitual trauma.

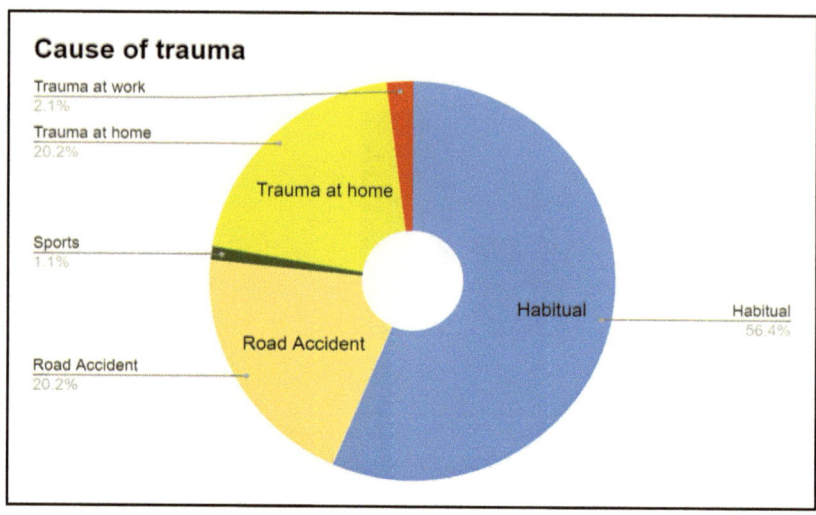

Figure 17. Distribution of patient according to the Cause of trauma

Characters of clavicle fracture

The results of this investigation clearly show that the incidence of type 15.2A is major. It was discovered that type 15.2A affects 48.9% of people. Type 15.2C was present in 29 individuals, or 30.9%. Type 15.3A in 9.6% patients,15.1A in 5.3%,15.3C in 3.2% and 15.1C in 2.1% patients was observed.

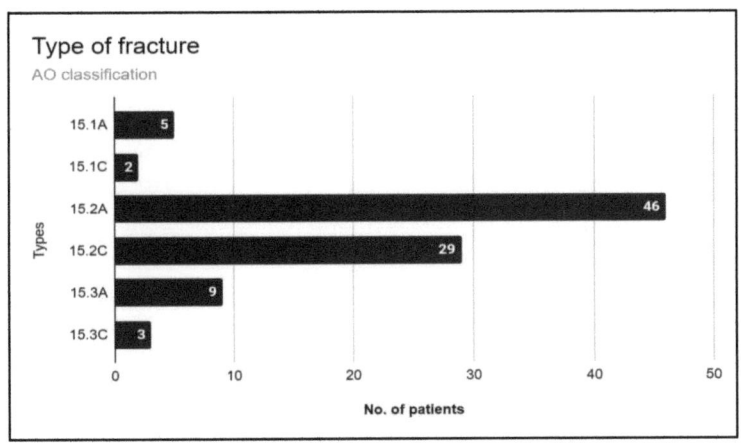

Fig 18. Distribution of the patients according to the type of fracture

From the data analyzed from the graph most clavicle fractures are 15.2A type(48.9%).

Localization – medial , middle, lateral

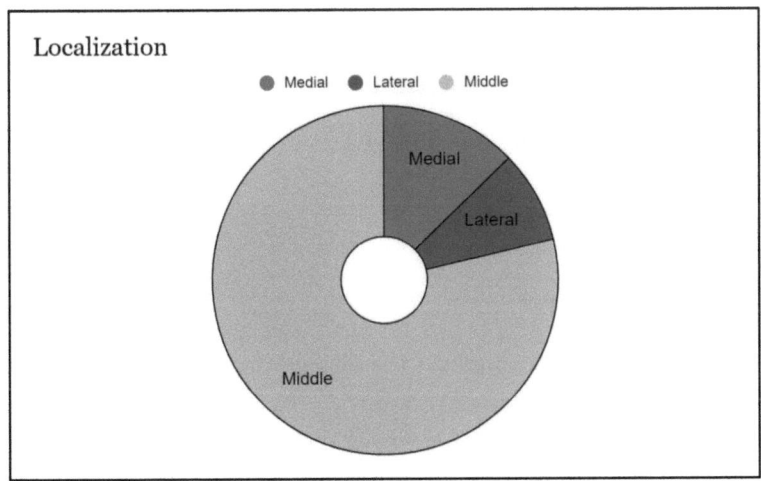

Fig 19. Distribution of the patients according to the localization of fracture

From the data analyzed from the graph the middle part of the clavicle is most common to be broken.

Side right-left

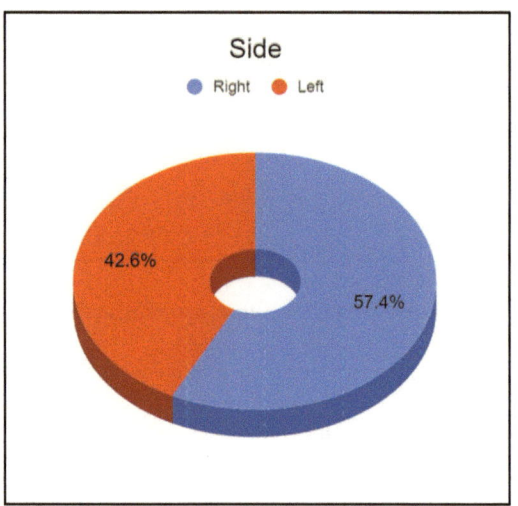

Fig 20.Distribution of the patients according to the localization side of fracture

We can observe from this graph that in general there is a slight majority for clavicle fractures to happen on the right side of the body.

Hospitalization and treatment

Based on the data analyzed from patients who arrived with a clavicle fracture, 79 individuals were discharged from the hospital in less than five days following their hospitalization. The majority of them arrived at the emergency room with minor wounds. Twelve patients were discharged in six to ten days and two patients took eleven to fifteen days. The length of hospital stay for clavicle fractures is primarily determined by a number of variables, including the extent of the damage, the patient's response to therapy post-operative complications, etc.

Period of hospitalization

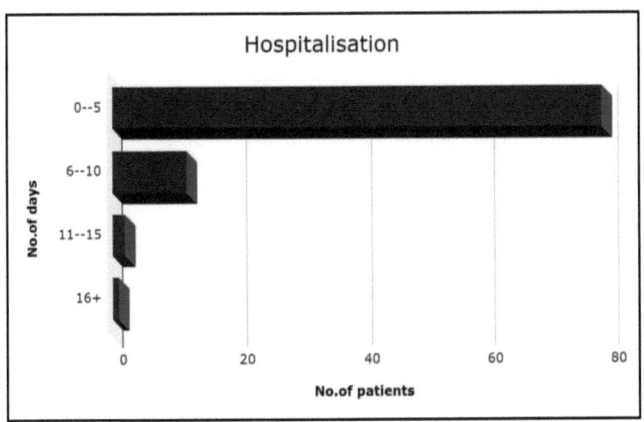

Fig 21. Distribution by days of hospitalization.

Trauma isolated-multiple

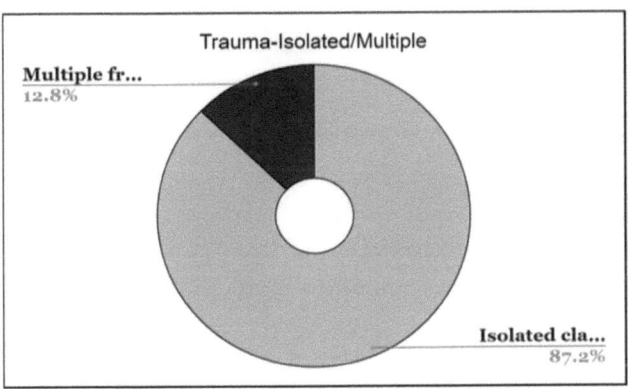

Fig 22. Distribution of the patients according to the multiple/isolated trauma

Clavicle fractures are mostly isolated fractures (87.2%), just a few fractures(12.8%) are associated with other fractures or dislocations. The most common associated injuries are fracture of the internal malleolus, acromio-clavicular dislocation, fracture of upper extremity of humerus and fracture of ribs.

Type of treatment

Surgical intervention was used to treat the majority of patients instead of a conservative strategy. It was discovered that patients who received plate osteosynthesis and open reduction were happier with the outcome and recovered more quickly.96.8% of patients underwent surgical treatment. Only 3.2% of all patients received conservative care, and they were primarily low-risk situations.

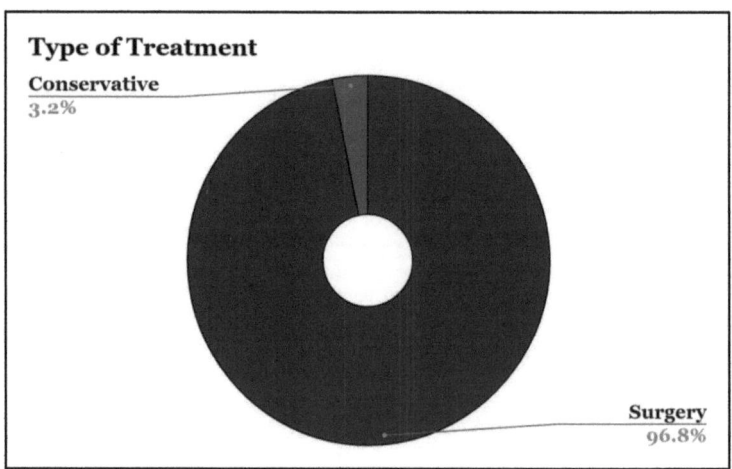

Fig 24.Type of treatment opted by patients

Postoperative complications

There are very few cases of postoperative complications of clavicle fractures. Injury of coracoclavicular ligaments can occur very rarely as a postoperative complication in clavicle fractures.

3. RESULTS AND DISCUSSION

3.1 Results and discussion

According to the study, clavicle fractures are most frequently discovered in individuals between the ages of 26 and 45 who are able to work. It also turns out that the faster a person recovers, the faster they are able to find job. The fact that the affected patients range in age from 26 to 45 on average supports the theory that clavicle fractures have a significant negative impact on the quality of life and capacity for self-care for traumatized individuals, particularly those from the working class.

We could discover that the patients with clavicle fractures spent an average of 3–4 days in the hospital, based on the study mentioned in the previous chapter. That is, a shorter hospital stays results in the following advantages: favorable effect on the patient's psychological state and positive societal impact. In this instance, the goal is to lower the cost of surgical treatments, which enables a higher level of attention to be paid to postoperative and immobilization manipulation and healing techniques.

Following the completion of this trial, the surgical approach to treating clavicle fractures was found to be especially important.

Compared to orthopedic treatment, surgical treatment for clavicle fractures assures a lower rate of complications. It also has a successful track record for treating difficult fractures such as comminuted fractures or osteoporosis-affected bone.

3.2 Clinical cases

Clinical case N1

Patient O, 40 years old. Visited to N1 Traumatology department of the Institute of Emergency Medicine on 14th April 2023.History of current illness: He falls from the scooter and hits a curb on the right side.(Trauma mechanism-direct).

Complaints: Soft tissue swelling, pathological clavicle deformity, impossibility of active movements of the right thoracic limb, pathological movements, bony crepitations.

X-ray of the clavicle (14/04/2023): Fracture of the right 1/3 lateral clavicle with displacement. Surgical intervention: Open reduction. Osteosynthesis of the clavicle on the right with plate and screws.

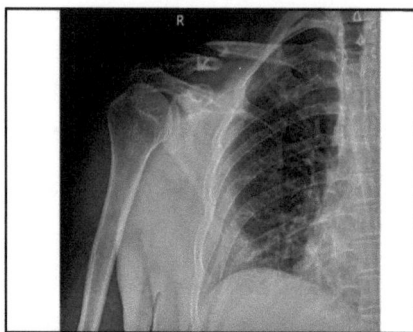 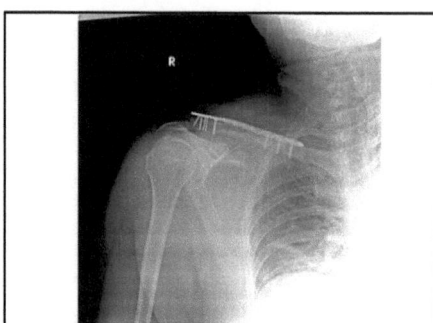

Figure 25. (a) X-ray of the clavicle: Fracture of the middle 1/3 of the clavicle(b) X-ray of the clavicle: Osteosynthesis of the clavicle on the right with plate and screws

Discharged on 18 April, 2023. The postoperative period without complications, discharged home in good condition.

Clinical case N2

Patient H, 79 years old. Visited to N1 Traumatology department of the Institute of Emergency Medicine on 24th February 2023.History of current illness: Trauma at home -falls in the left shoulder(Trauma mechanism-direct).

Complaints: pain in the region of the left clavicle, functional impotence, pain, edema, deformity, bony crepitation in the region are detected. right clavicle, functional impotence of the right shoulder joint.

X-ray of the clavicle (24/02/2023): Fracture of the sternal portion of the left clavicle with displacement. Anterior dislocation of the left humerus

Surgical intervention: Open reduction. Osteosynthesis of the clavicle on the left with plate and screws.

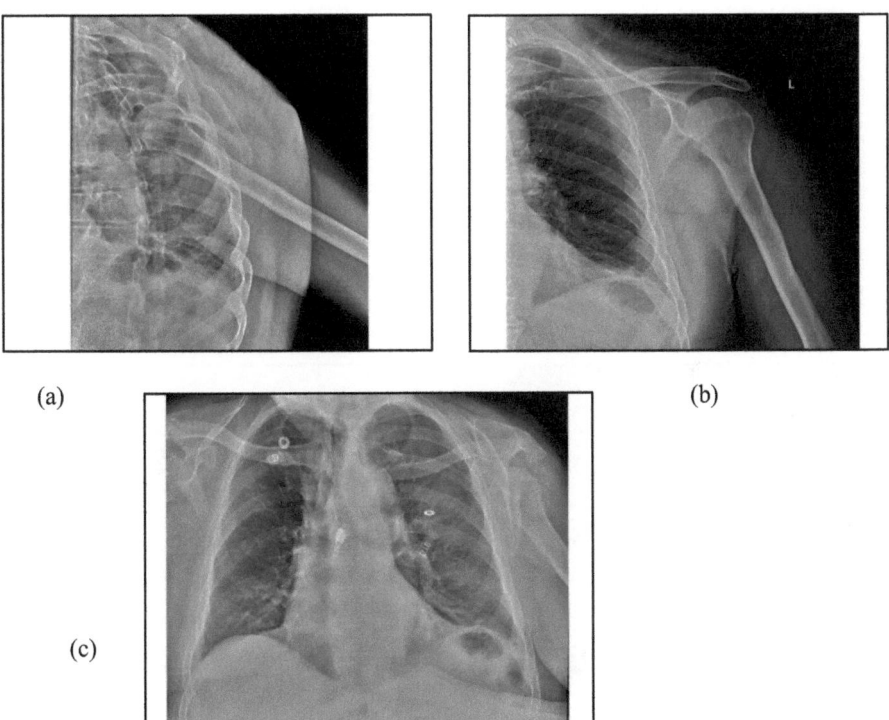

(a)

(b)

(c)

Figure 26. (a) X-ray of the clavicle: Anterior dislocation of the left humerus

(b) X-ray of the clavicle: After putting the humerus in place

(c)X-ray of the clavicle: Fracture of the sternal portion of the left clavicle with displacement

Discharged on 27 February, 2023. The postoperative period without complications, discharged home in good condition.

Clinical case N3

Patient L, 31 years old. Visited to N1 Traumatology department of the Institute of Emergency Medicine on 16th May 2023.History of current illness: trauma in the Czech Republic, fell from a tree on the left shoulder on 09.05.2023, was assisted in the Czech Republic, Delibet rings were applied. On 15.05.2023 he went to the family doctor. On 16.05.2023, came to IMSP IMU

Complaints: pain in the clavicle region goes away, functional impotence. Left thoracic limb immobilized in Delbet rings, unstable. Edema, post-traumatic ecchymosis of the clavicle region on the left. Limitation of active and passive movements in the left shoulder joint, bony crepitus and pain when palpating the left clavicle.

X-ray of the clavicle (16/05/2023):   Fracture of the left clavicle in the average 1/3 without displacement with metal fixation.

Surgical intervention: Open reduction. Osteosynthesis of the comminuted fracture of the left clavicle with plate and screws

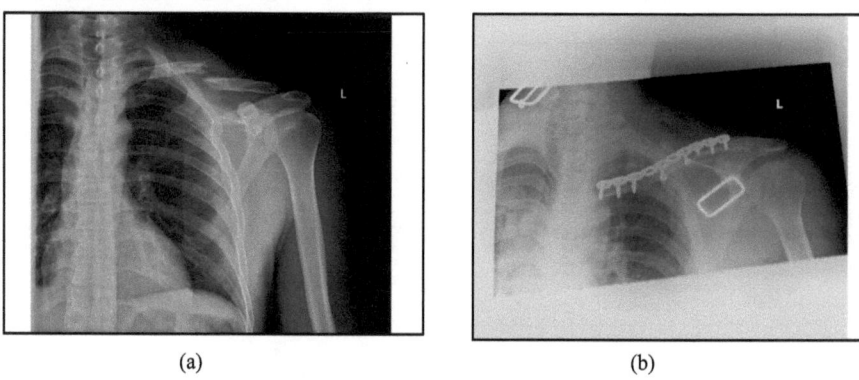

(a)   (b)

Figure 27. (a) X-ray of the clavicle: Fracture of the left clavicle in the average ⅓

(b) X-ray of the clavicle: Osteosynthesis of the comminuted fracture of the left clavicle with plate and screws

Discharged on 22 May, 2023. The postoperative period without complications, discharged home in good condition.

CONCLUSIONS

1. In the traumatology department, fractures of the clavicle are a common injury. These injuries can significantly impair a patient's capacity for self-care and self-service, emphasizing the societal significance of appropriate treatment options.

2. Our research indicates that men (77.7%) of working age (21–60 years) make up the bulk of patients with clavicle fractures, and a quicker healing time may improve their quality of life and capacity to resume work.

3. 96.8% of patients received ORIF surgery. Many clavicle fractures are treated conservatively, but these patients don't need admission to the hospital.

4. Compared to conservative treatment, surgical treatment has a lower rate of complications (2%) and a shorter hospital stay (1–5 days) for treating clavicle fractures.

BIBLIOGRAPHY

1. Allman F. L. Fractures and ligamentous injuries of the clavicle and its articulation. In: The Journal of Bone & Joint Surgery. 1967, nr.49(4), p.774-784.

2. Aminian A., Giotakis N., Abbasian M., & Ebrahimi H. Management of complications following clavicle fracture surgery. In: Journal of Orthopaedic Surgery and Research, 2013, nr.7(1), p.1-7.

3. Andermahr J, Jubel A, Elsner A, Johann J, Prokop A, Rehm KE, Koebke J. Anatomy of the clavicle and the intramedullary nailing of midclavicular fractures. Clin Anat. 2007;20(1):48–56

4. Anakwenze O. A., Zuckerman J. D. Classifications in brief: Allman classification of clavicle fractures. In: Clinical Orthopaedics and Related Research, 2014, nr. 472(11), p.3618-3622.

5. Bahrs C., Stojicevic T., Blumenstock G., Brorson S., Badke, A., Stockle, U. Trends in epidemiology and patho-anatomical pattern of clavicle fractures: A study of 452 cases. In: Archives of Orthopaedic and Trauma Surgery, 2014, nr. 134(3), p. 405-412.

6. Bhatia D. N., de Beer J., Van Rooyen, K. Diagnosis and management of acromioclavicular joint injuries. In: Current Reviews in Musculoskeletal Medicine, 2013, nr.6(1), p.71-77.

7. Bozkurt M., Can F., & Kirdemir V. Neurovascular complications of clavicle fractures: Rare but dangerous. In: Acta Orthopaedica et Traumatologica Turcica, 2015, nr.46(3), p.207-211.

8. Canadian Orthopaedic Trauma Society. Nonoperative treatment compared with plate fixation of displaced midshaft clavicular fractures: a multicenter, randomized clinical trial. In: The Journal of Bone & Joint Surgery, 2007, nr. 89(1), 1-10.

9. Chen, C. E., Hsu, S. Y., Lin, J. H., Huang, C. I. Ultrasound evaluation of clavicle fractures. In: American Journal of Emergency Medicine, 2011, nr. 29(9), p.1172-1175.

10. Egol, K. A., Koval, K. J., Zuckerman, J. D., & Handbook of Fractures, Third Edition. Fractures of the clavicle. 2010, Wolters Kluwer/Lippincott Williams & Wilkins, p.320.

11. Eygendaal, D., Kraan, G. A., & van Lieshout, E. M.. Surgical treatment of clavicle fractures: a review of the literature. In: Bulletin of the NYU Hospital for Joint Diseases, 2013, nr. 71(1), p.59-65.

12. Frima H.,van Heijl M.,Michelitsch C.,van der Meijden O.,Beeres F.J.P.,Houwert R.M.,Sommer C. Clavicle fractures in adults; current concepts.Eur J Trauma Emerg Surg. 2020; 46: 519-529

13. Goldberg, J. A., Viglione, W., Kelly, J. D., Akelman, E. Nerve injury and recovery after lateral clavicle fractures: A clinicopathologic study. In: The Journal of Shoulder and Elbow Surgery, 1997, nr. 6(4), p. 287-292.

14. Goss, T. P. Double disruptions of the superior shoulder suspensory complex.In: The Journal of Orthopaedic Trauma, 1998, nr. 12(4), p. 337-341.

15. Hill, J. M., McGuire, M. H., & Crosby, L. A. (1997). Closed treatment of displaced middle-third fractures of the clavicle gives poor results. The Journal of Bone & Joint Surgery, 79(4), 537-539.

16. Houwert, R. M., Wijdicks, F. J., Steins Bisschop, C. N., Verhofstad, M. H., & Van Lieshout, E. M. (2016). Acute neurovascular complications in displaced clavicle fractures: an analysis of 107 consecutive fractures. International Orthopaedics, 40(9), 1951-1954

17. Jupiter, J. B., & Leffert, R. D. (1990). Nonunion of the clavicle. The Journal of Bone & Joint Surgery, 72(3), 328-337.

18. Kelly, J. D., & A review of operative management of clavicle fractures. (2007). Bulletin of the NYU Hospital for Joint Diseases, 65(1), 47-53.

19. Kettler, M., Schieker, M., Braunstein, V., & Mutschler, W. (2012). Flexible intramedullary nailing of clavicular midshaft fractures: a matched-pair study. The Journal of Bone & Joint Surgery, 94(8), 678-686.

20. Lenza, M., Buchbinder, R., Johnston, R. V., Belloti, J. C., & Faloppa, F. (2013). Surgical versus conservative interventions for treating fractures of the middle third of the clavicle. Cochrane Database of Systematic Reviews, (6).

21. Luo TD, Ashraf A, Larson AN, Stans AA, Shaughnessy WJ, McIntosh AL. Complications in the treatment of adolescent clavicle fractures. Orthopedics. 2015 Apr;38(4):e287-91.

22. Mehta, V., & Bain, G. I. (2013). The anatomy of the clavicle: Its surgical significance. Clinical Anatomy, 26(3), 345-357.

23. McKee RC, Whelan DB, Schemitsch EH, McKee MD. Operative versus nonoperative care of displaced midshaft clavicular fractures: a meta-analysis of randomized clinical trials. J Bone Jt Surg Am. 2012;94(8):675–84.

24. Mohan, R., Ramesh, B., & Pai, S. B. (2012). The role of radiography and ultrasonography in the diagnosis of clavicular fractures. Journal of Clinical Imaging Science, 2(1), 59.

25. Murthi, A. M., Vosburgh, C. L., & Neviaser, R. J. (2005). The incidence of anomalous coracoclavicular joints. Journal of Shoulder and Elbow Surgery, 14(5), 534-537.

26. Muthusamy, S., & Kalyanasundaram, D. (2019). A study on morphometric analysis of clavicle in South Indian population. Journal of Clinical and Diagnostic Research, 13(2), AC01-AC03.

27. Neer, C. S. (1960). Fractures of the clavicle. The Journal of Bone & Joint Surgery, 42(3), 476-484.

28. Neer CS. Fractures of the distal third of the clavicle. Clin Orthop Relat Res. 1968 May-Jun;58:43-50.

29. Nordqvist, A., & Petersson, C. (1994). The incidence of fractures of the clavicle. Clinical Orthopaedics and Related Research, (300), 127-132.

30. Nordqvist, A., Petersson, C., & Redlund-Johnell, I. (1998). The natural course of lateral clavicle fracture: 15 (11-21) year follow-up of 110 cases. Acta Orthopaedica Scandinavica, 69(5), 48-50.

31. Nowak, J., Holgersson, M., & Larsson, S. (2005). Sequelae from clavicular fractures are common: a prospective study of 222 patients. Acta Orthopaedica, 76(4), 496-502.

32. Postacchini, F., Gumina, S., De Santis, P., Albo, F., & Ferrara, A. (2002). Epidemiology of clavicle fractures. Journal of Shoulder and Elbow Surgery, 11(5), 452-456.

33. Ropars M, Thomazeau H, Huten D. Clavicle fractures. Orthop Traumatol Surg Res. 2017 Feb;103(1S):S53-S59.

34. Robinson CM, Goudie EB, Murray IR, Jenkins PJ, Ahktar MA, Read EO, et al. Open reduction and plate fixation versus nonoperative treatment for displaced midshaft clavicular fractures: a multicenter, randomized, controlled trial. J Bone Jt Surg Am. 2013;95(17):1576–84.

35. Robinson, C. M., & Akhtar, M. A. (2018). Fractures of the clavicle. In Bucholz and Heckman's fracture treatment (pp. 1137-1162). Wolters Kluwer.

36. Robinson, C. M., & Court-Brown, C. M. (2006). The management of midshaft clavicle fractures: A comparison of plating and intramedullary nailing. The Journal of Bone & Joint Surgery, 88(1), 106-112.

37. "Rockwood and Green's Fractures in Adults" edited by Charles A. Rockwood Jr., Paul Tornetta III, and James R. Krieg (2019)

38. Rowe CR. An atlas of anatomy and treatment of midclavicular fractures. Clin Orthop Relat Res. 1968;58:29–42.

39. Sanders, R., & Swiontkowski, M. (2003). Treatment of diaphyseal fractures of the humerus and the clavicle. Instructional Course Lectures, 52, 131-143.

40. Sidhu VS, Hermans D, Duckworth DG. The operative outcomes of displaced medial-end clavicle fractures. J Shoulder Elbow Surg. 2015;24(11):1728–34.

41. Skedros, J. G., & Hunt, K. J. (2004). The association of clavicular facet morphology with the occurrence of midshaft clavicular fractures. The American Journal of Sports Medicine, 32(2), 478-483.

42. Slongo, T., Audige, L., Clavert, P., & Lutz, N. (2015). AO pediatric comprehensive classification of long bone fractures (PCCF). European Journal of Pediatric Surgery, 25(2), 143-154.

43. Smekal, V., Irenberger, A., Attal, R. E., Oberladstätter, J., Krappinger, D., & Kralinger, F. S. (2009). Elastic stable intramedullary nailing is the treatment of choice for midshaft clavicular fracture in adults: results in 142 patients. Injury, 40(12), 1312-1316.

44. Society COT. Nonoperative treatment compared with plate fixation of displaced midshaft clavicular fractures. A multicenter, randomized clinical trial. J Bone Jt Surg Am. 2007;89(1):1–10.

45. Standring, S. (Ed.). (2016). Gray's anatomy: The anatomical basis of clinical practice (41st ed.). Elsevier Health Sciences.

46. Stanley, D., Trowbridge, E. A., & Norris, S. H. (1988). The mechanism of clavicular fracture: A clinical and biomechanical analysis. Journal of Bone and Joint Surgery, 70(2), 233-237.

47. Tamaoki, M. J., & Belloti, J. C. (2015). Treatment of clavicle fractures: current concepts review. Revista Brasileira de Ortopedia, 50(1), 9-16.

48. Venclauskas, L., Siloveckas, R., Valaikaite, R., Cekanauskas, E., & Malinauskas, M. (2016). Epidemiology of clavicle

fractures in Lithuania in 2011-2013. Medicina, 52(1), 29-34.

49. Wiesel B, Nagda S, Mehta S, Churchill R. Management of Midshaft Clavicle Fractures in Adults. J Am Acad Orthop Surg. 2018 Nov 15;26(22):e468-e476.

50. Williams, G. R., Nguyen, V. D., Rockwood, C. A. Jr, & Bigliani, L. U. (1989). A classification system for injuries to the acromioclavicular joint. The Journal of Bone & Joint Surgery, 71(6), 939-943.

51. Wijdicks, C. A., Wheeler, D. L., & Dvorak, J. (2012). Biomechanical evaluation of clavicle fracture plating techniques: Does malunion impact failure loads? Journal of Orthopaedic Trauma, 26(4), 244-249.

52. Zlowodzki, M., Zelle, B. A., Cole, P. A., Jeray, K., McKee, M. D., & Evidence-Based Orthopedic Trauma Working Group. (2005). Treatment of acute midshaft clavicle fractures: systematic review of 2144 fractures: On behalf of the Evidence-Based Orthopaedic Trauma Working Group. Journal of Orthopaedic Trauma, 19(7), 504-507.

Image References

53.https://surgeryreference.aofoundation.org/orthopedic-trauma/adult-trauma/ clavicle-fractures

54.https://doldmd.com/shoulder-and-elbow/clavicle-collar-bone-fracture/

55.https://radiopaedia.org/articles/clavicular-fracture

56.https://www.kaplinsportsmed.com/shoulder-orthopedic-sports-medicine-specialist - cherry-hill-mt-laurel-moorestown.html

57.https://www.perthortho.com.au/extra-information/shoulder-anatomy